Stretching Exercises For Seniors over 60

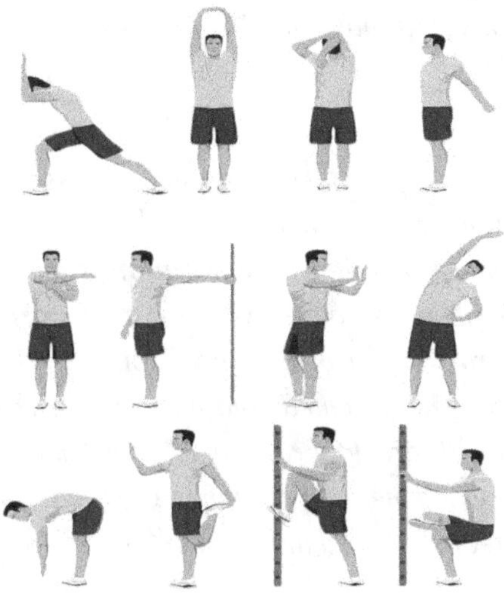

*Gentle Moves for a Healthier You to Stay
Flexible and Active in Your Golden Age*

Diana E. Allison

Table of Content

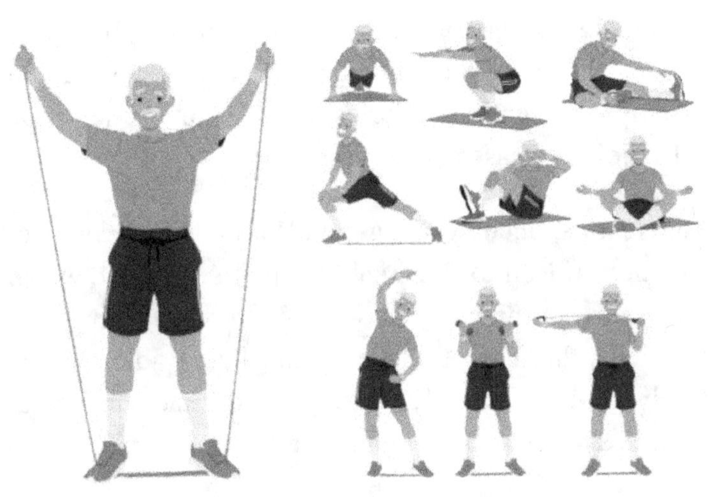

Introduction

Welcome to a journey of renewed vitality and flexibility. As we grow older, keeping an active lifestyle becomes increasingly important. Stretching exercises are not just about staying fit; they are about enhancing your quality of life, preventing injuries, and enjoying everyday activities with ease and comfort.

For seniors, incorporating regular stretching into your routine can lead to remarkable benefits. Imagine waking up each morning with less stiffness, feeling more energetic throughout the day, and being able to move freely and confidently. These gentle movements are designed to help you achieve just that.

In this guide, we will explore a variety of stretching exercises tailored specifically for your needs. Whether you're a seasoned exerciser or new to fitness, these stretches are simple, safe, and highly effective. Our goal is to make you feel stronger, more flexible, and ready to embrace every moment of your golden years.

Let's embark on this path to better health together, and discover how a few minutes of stretching each day can transform your life. Get ready to feel more youthful, vibrant, and active than ever before!

Importance of Stretching for Seniors

Stretching plays a pivotal role in the health and well-being of seniors, offering a multitude of benefits that enhance daily life and overall vitality. As we age, our muscles naturally lose elasticity, and joints become stiffer, making movement more challenging. Incorporating regular stretching into your routine can counteract these effects and provide significant advantages:

1. **Maintaining Flexibility**: Stretching helps to improve and maintain flexibility in muscles and joints. This increased flexibility translates into better range of motion, allowing seniors to perform daily activities with greater ease and comfort.

2. **Improving Posture**: Good posture is essential for balance and reducing the risk of falls, which can be particularly detrimental for seniors. Stretching exercises promote proper alignment of the spine and muscles, contributing to better posture and stability.

3. **Reducing Muscle Tension and Soreness:** Stretching helps to alleviate muscle tension and reduce the likelihood of muscle soreness after physical activity or prolonged periods of sitting or standing. This can enhance mobility and decrease discomfort.

4. **Enhancing Blood Circulation:** Engaging in stretching movements stimulates blood flow to muscles and joints, promoting better circulation

throughout the body. Improved circulation contributes to faster healing of injuries and better overall cardiovascular health.

5. **Increasing Energy Levels:** Regular stretching can boost energy levels by increasing blood flow and oxygen delivery to tissues. This can result in feeling more invigorated and less fatigued throughout the day.

6. **Preventing Injuries**: Flexible muscles and joints are less prone to injuries such as strains, sprains, and muscle pulls. Stretching helps to prepare the body for physical activities and reduces the risk of injury during exercise or daily tasks.

7. **Enhancing Mental Well-being**: Stretching exercises can have a positive impact on mental health by promoting relaxation, reducing stress levels, and improving overall mood. This holistic approach to fitness can contribute to a better quality of life in senior years.

Incorporating a variety of stretching exercises into your daily routine, tailored to your individual needs and abilities, can significantly enhance your physical and mental well-being as you navigate the golden years. Embrace the benefits of stretching and enjoy a more active, fulfilling life with improved mobility and vitality.

Benefits of Regular Stretching

Regular stretching offers a wide array of benefits that contribute to both physical health and overall well-being, especially for seniors. Here are the key advantages:

1. **Improved Flexibility and Range of Motion:** Stretching exercises help to lengthen muscles and increase flexibility in joints, allowing for improved range of motion. This flexibility is essential for performing daily activities with ease and reducing the risk of injury.

2. **Enhanced Muscle Function**: Stretching promotes better muscle coordination and balance, which are crucial for maintaining stability and preventing falls, a significant concern for seniors.

3. **Reduced Muscle Tension and Soreness:** Stretching relaxes tense muscles and alleviates stiffness, providing relief from discomfort often associated with aging, prolonged sitting, or physical activity.

4. **Better Posture and Alignment:** Stretching helps to correct muscular imbalances, improve posture, and align the spine properly. This can reduce

strain on the back and neck, enhancing overall body mechanics.

5. **Improved Circulation:** Stretching increases blood flow to muscles and joints, promoting better circulation throughout the body. Enhanced circulation supports faster recovery from injuries and contributes to cardiovascular health.

6. **Stress Relief and Relaxation:** Engaging in stretching exercises promotes relaxation by releasing tension stored in muscles. This can lower stress levels, improve mood, and contribute to better mental well-being.

7. **Prevention of Injuries:** Flexible muscles and tendons are less likely to be strained or injured during physical activities or daily tasks. Regular stretching prepares the body for movement and reduces the risk of muscle strains, sprains, and other injuries.

8. **Enhanced Performance in Physical Activities:** Increased flexibility and improved muscle function translate into better performance in sports, recreational activities, and everyday tasks, allowing seniors to maintain an active lifestyle.

9. **Support for Joint Health**: Stretching helps to maintain joint health by preserving the lubricating synovial fluid and preventing stiffness that can lead to arthritis or other joint-related issues.

10. **Promotion of Longevity and Quality of Life**: By improving flexibility, reducing muscle tension, and supporting overall physical health, regular stretching can contribute to a higher quality of life and promote independence as individuals age.

Regular stretching is not just a simple routine; it's a pathway to maintaining and enhancing your physical and mental well-being as you age. The benefits of stretching exercises for seniors are profound and far-reaching, from improving flexibility and range of motion to reducing muscle tension and enhancing overall posture and balance.

Chapter 1: Safety Tips

Warming Up

Warming up before stretching is essential to prepare your muscles and joints for activity, reducing the risk of injury and enhancing the effectiveness of your stretching routine. Follow these tips to ensure a safe and effective warm-up:

1. **Start with Light Aerobic Activity:** Begin your warm-up with 5-10 minutes of light aerobic exercise such as walking, marching in place, or cycling on a stationary bike. This increases your heart rate and blood flow to your muscles.

2. **Focus on Dynamic Movements**: Incorporate dynamic movements that mimic the motions you'll be doing during stretching. For example, arm circles, leg swings, or gentle twists can help loosen up joints and increase flexibility.

3. **Gradually Increase Intensity:** Progressively increase the intensity of your warm-up activities.

Start with gentle movements and gradually move into larger range-of-motion exercises as your muscles begin to feel more limber.

4. **Include Specific Joint Movements**: Pay attention to areas that will be targeted during your stretching routine. Move your joints through their full range of motion to lubricate the joint capsules and prepare them for stretching.

5. **Listen to Your Body**: Pay attention to how your body feels during the warm-up. It's normal to feel a slight increase in temperature and mild sweating, but you should not experience pain or discomfort. If you do, adjust your intensity or technique.

6. **Stay Hydrated**: Drink water before and after your warm-up to stay hydrated. Proper hydration supports muscle function and helps regulate body temperature during exercise.

By incorporating these warming-up tips into your stretching routine, you'll ensure that your muscles are adequately prepared for activity, reducing the risk of strains or injuries. A proper warm-up not only enhances the effectiveness of your stretches but also sets the foundation for a safe and enjoyable exercise session.

Proper Technique

Maintaining proper technique during stretching exercises is crucial to maximize benefits and prevent injury, especially for seniors. Follow these guidelines to ensure safe and effective stretching:

1. **Warm Up First:** Always begin with a gentle warm-up to increase blood flow to your muscles and prepare them for stretching. This helps reduce muscle stiffness and improves flexibility.

2. **Start Slowly**: Begin each stretch slowly and gently without bouncing or jerking. Ease into the stretch until you feel mild tension, stopping before you feel pain.

3. **Hold Each Stretch**: Hold each stretch for 15-30 seconds, or longer if comfortable, to allow your muscles time to relax and lengthen. Avoid holding your breath; instead, breathe deeply and steadily.

4. **Focus on the Muscle Group**: Concentrate on the specific muscle group you're targeting with each stretch. Visualize the muscle lengthening and gradually increasing flexibility.

5. **Avoid Overstretching**: Stretch to the point of mild discomfort, but never to the point of pain. Overstretching can cause muscle strains or other injuries, especially in older adults.

6. **Use Proper Alignment**: Maintain proper body alignment during each stretch. For example, keep your spine neutral and shoulders relaxed when stretching the neck and upper back.

7. **Modify as Needed**: If you have joint problems or specific health concerns, modify stretches to accommodate your needs. Consult with a healthcare professional or physical therapist for personalized advice.

8. **Stay Consistent:** Incorporate stretching into your daily routine to maintain and improve flexibility over time. Consistency is key to reaping the long-term benefits of stretching exercises.

By following these guidelines for proper technique, you can safely and effectively incorporate stretching into your fitness regimen. Remember, stretching should feel good and contribute to your overall well-being without causing discomfort or pain.

Listening to Your Body

Listening to your body is essential during stretching exercises, particularly for seniors, to ensure safety and maximize the benefits of your routine. Here are key considerations to help you tune into your body's signals:

1. **Respect Your Limits:** Understand that everyone's flexibility and range of motion vary. Respect your body's current capabilities and avoid pushing yourself beyond comfortable limits.

2. **Pay Attention to Sensations**: During stretching, pay attention to sensations in your muscles and joints. Mild discomfort or tension is normal, but sharp pain or excessive discomfort indicates you should ease off the stretch.

3. **Breathe Mindfully:** Use your breath as a guide. Breathe deeply and rhythmically during stretches to help relax your muscles and enhance the effectiveness of each stretch.

4. **Modify as Needed**: If a stretch feels too intense or causes pain, modify it to a more comfortable position or try a different stretch that targets the

same muscle group. There's no one-size-fits-all approach, so find what works best for you.

5. **Be Patient and Gentle**: Allow yourself time to gradually improve flexibility. Avoid sudden or forceful movements that could strain muscles or joints. Gentle, steady progress is key to long-term success.

6. **Listen to Feedback:** Your body provides feedback through sensations of stretching, tightness, or relaxation. Learn to interpret these signals to adjust your stretching routine accordingly.

7. **Stay Hydrated:** Maintain proper hydration before and after stretching exercises. Dehydration can contribute to muscle stiffness and cramping, affecting your ability to stretch effectively.

8. **Consult a Professional:** If you have chronic pain, specific health conditions, or concerns about stretching exercises, consult with a healthcare professional or physical therapist for personalized guidance.

By listening to your body and honoring its signals during stretching exercises, you can cultivate a safe and effective routine that supports your overall health and well-being. Adjust your stretches as needed, stay mindful of your body's responses, and enjoy the benefits of improved flexibility and mobility.

When to Seek Medical Advice

While stretching exercises offer numerous benefits for seniors, it's important to be mindful of your body's responses and seek medical advice when necessary. Here are situations where consulting a healthcare professional is recommended:

1. **Persistent Pain:** If you experience persistent or sharp pain during or after stretching exercises, especially in specific joints or muscles, it may indicate an underlying issue such as arthritis, tendonitis, or a muscle strain.

2. **Decreased Range of Motion:** If you notice a sudden or gradual decrease in your range of motion despite regular stretching, it could be a sign of joint stiffness, inflammation, or other musculoskeletal conditions that require evaluation.

3. **Difficulty Performing Daily Activities**: If stiffness or pain from stretching exercises interferes with your ability to perform daily activities such as walking, climbing stairs, or getting up from a chair, it's important to discuss these symptoms with a healthcare provider.

4. **New Symptoms**: If you develop new symptoms such as swelling, numbness, tingling, or weakness in muscles or joints after stretching, it may indicate an injury or nerve-related issue that requires medical attention.

5. **Pre-existing Medical Conditions:** If you have pre-existing medical conditions such as osteoporosis, osteoarthritis, cardiovascular disease, or diabetes, consult with your doctor before starting a new stretching routine to ensure it's safe and appropriate for your health status.

6. **Recent Surgery or Injury:** If you've undergone recent surgery or are recovering from an injury, seek guidance from your healthcare provider or physical therapist before engaging in stretching exercises to avoid complications or setbacks in your recovery.

7. **Persistent Joint Swelling**: If you experience persistent swelling or inflammation in your joints, particularly after stretching exercises, it may indicate an underlying joint condition that requires medical evaluation and treatment.

8. **Unexplained Fatigue or Weakness:** If you feel unusually fatigued or weak during or after stretching exercises, it could be a sign of overexertion, dehydration, or an underlying medical issue that warrants medical assessment.

By monitoring your body's responses and seeking medical advice when necessary, you can ensure that your stretching routine supports your overall health and well-being without compromising safety. Your healthcare provider can provide personalized recommendations and guidance to help you achieve optimal results from your stretching exercises.

Chapter 2: Upper Body Stretches

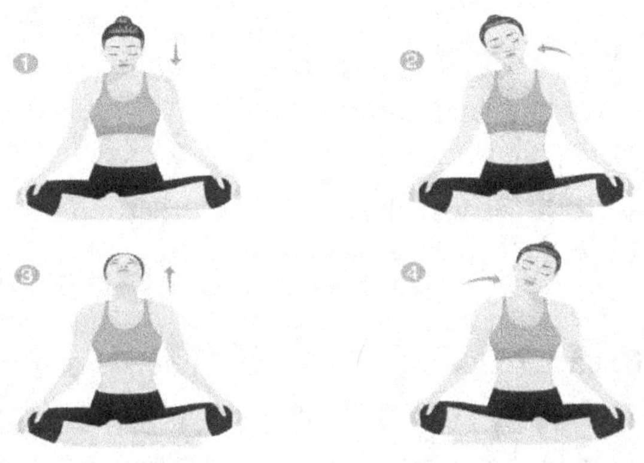

Neck Stretch

The neck stretch is a simple yet effective exercise to alleviate tension and improve flexibility in the neck and upper shoulders. Follow these steps for a safe and effective neck stretch:

1. **Sit or Stand Tall**: Maintain good posture with your shoulders relaxed and spine straight.

2. **Slowly Tilt Your Head:** Gently tilt your head to one side, bringing your ear towards your

shoulder. Avoid lifting or rotating your shoulder;
keep it relaxed.

3. **Hold the Stretch**: Hold the position for 15-30
   seconds, feeling a gentle stretch along the side of
   your neck and shoulder.

4. **Switch Sides:** Return your head to the center
   position and repeat the stretch on the opposite
   side.
5. **Breathe Deeply:** Take slow, deep breaths as you
   hold each stretch to help relax the muscles and
   deepen the stretch.

6. **Repeat as Needed:** You can perform the neck
   stretch several times throughout the day,
   especially if you spend long periods sitting at a
   desk or computer.

Safety Tips:
- **Avoid Overstretching:** Only stretch to the point
  where you feel a gentle pull; do not force the
  stretch or cause pain.

- **Be Gentle**: The neck is sensitive, so be gentle
  and gradual in your movements.

- **Consult a Professional:** If you have neck pain or a history of neck injuries, consult with a healthcare provider or physical therapist before performing neck stretches.

Incorporating the neck stretch into your daily routine can help alleviate stiffness, improve posture, and reduce discomfort in the neck and shoulders, promoting overall neck health and well-being.

Shoulder Stretch

The shoulder stretch helps to improve flexibility and relieve tension in the shoulders and upper back. Follow these steps to perform a safe and effective shoulder stretch:

1. **Stand Tall or Sit Comfortably**: Maintain good posture with your spine straight and shoulders relaxed.

2. **Reach Across Your Body**: Extend one arm across your chest at shoulder height, keeping it straight but not locked.

3. **Use Your Opposite Hand:** Use your opposite hand to gently pull your extended arm towards

your chest. Avoid pulling too hard; the stretch should be gentle and comfortable.

4. **Hold the Stretch**: Hold the position for 15-30 seconds, feeling a stretch in the back of your shoulder and upper arm.

5. **Switch Sides**: Release the stretch and repeat with the opposite arm.

6. **Breathe Deeply**: Take slow, deep breaths as you hold each stretch to relax your muscles and deepen the stretch.

7. **Repeat as Needed**: You can perform the shoulder stretch multiple times throughout the day, especially if you experience tightness or discomfort in your shoulders.

Safety Tips:
- **Avoid Jerking Movements:** Perform the stretch with slow, controlled movements to prevent strain or injury.

- **Modify as Needed:** If you have shoulder problems or limitations in range of motion, adjust the stretch to a comfortable position or consult with a healthcare provider.

- **Listen to Your Body:** Stop the stretch if you feel pain or discomfort beyond a gentle stretch sensation.

Incorporate this shoulder stretch into your daily routine as part of a holistic approach to maintaining mobility and comfort in your upper body. It's an essential exercise within our book's framework, designed to enhance overall physical well-being and promote a healthier lifestyle in your golden years.

Chest Stretch

To perform a safe and effective chest stretch, follow these steps:

1. **Prepare:** Stand tall with your feet hip-width apart or sit upright on a chair with good posture, ensuring your shoulders are relaxed and your spine is straight.

2. **Interlace Your Fingers:** Clasp your hands together behind your back, palms facing inward, or interlace your fingers in front of your body at chest level.

3. **Open Your Chest:** Slowly squeeze your shoulder blades together and gently lift your arms if clasped behind your back, or gently push your interlaced hands forward while keeping your arms straight. This action will open up your chest and shoulders.

4. **Hold the Stretch**: Hold the position for 15-30 seconds, feeling a gentle stretch across the front of your chest and shoulders. Avoid arching your back excessively; keep your spine neutral.

5. **Breathe Deeply**: Take deep, slow breaths as you hold the stretch. Inhale through your nose, expanding your chest, and exhale slowly through your mouth to enhance relaxation.

6. **Release and Repeat:** Slowly release the stretch and relax your arms. Repeat the stretch 2-3 times, adjusting your hand position slightly each time to ensure a thorough stretch.

Safety Tips:
- **Avoid Overstretching:** Stretch to the point of mild tension or discomfort, but never to the point of pain.

- **Maintain Control**: Perform the stretch with slow, controlled movements to prevent strain or injury.
- **Modify as Needed:** If you have shoulder or neck issues, adjust the hand position or consult with a healthcare professional for alternative stretches.

Incorporating this chest stretch into your regular routine can help improve posture, reduce stiffness in the chest and shoulders, and enhance overall upper body flexibility.

Chapter 3: Body Stretches

Hamstring Stretch

The hamstring stretch is a crucial exercise to enhance flexibility and improve lower body mobility. Follow these steps to perform the hamstring stretch effectively:

1. **Sit or Stand Comfortably:** Begin by sitting on the edge of a chair or standing with your feet hip-width apart and knees slightly bent to maintain stability.

2. **Extend One Leg Forward:** Extend one leg straight out in front of you with your heel on the ground and toes pointing upwards. Keep your back straight and shoulders relaxed.

3. **Hinge at the Hips:** Slowly lean forward from your hips, keeping your back straight, and reach towards your extended foot. Avoid rounding your back.

4. **Feel the Stretch:** You should feel a gentle stretch along the back of your thigh (hamstring). Adjust the intensity by leaning further forward or pulling your toes towards you.

5. **Hold the Stretch**: Hold the position for 15-30 seconds, breathing deeply and evenly throughout.

6. **Switch Legs**: Release the stretch and switch to the other leg, repeating the same steps.

7. **Repeat as Needed**: Perform the hamstring stretch 2-3 times on each leg to improve flexibility and reduce tension in the hamstrings.

Safety Tips:
- **Avoid Bouncing:** Perform the stretch with slow, controlled movements. Bouncing can strain the muscles and lead to injury.

- **Modify as Needed**: If you have difficulty reaching your foot, use a towel or strap around your foot to gently pull towards you.

- **Consult a Professional:** If you have chronic knee or back problems, consult with a healthcare provider or physical therapist before performing hamstring stretches.

Incorporating the hamstring stretch into your routine can help maintain and improve lower body flexibility, making everyday activities more comfortable and enjoyable.

Calf Stretch

The calf stretch is a beneficial exercise to enhance flexibility in the lower legs and improve mobility. Follow these steps to perform the calf stretch effectively:

1. **Find a Stable Surface:** Stand facing a wall or sturdy object for support. Place your hands on the wall or hold onto the back of a chair for balance.

2. **Step Back:** Take a step back with one foot, keeping both feet flat on the ground and toes pointing forward.

3. **Straighten Your Back Leg:** Keep your back leg straight with the heel firmly planted on the ground.

4. **Lean Forward:** Slowly lean forward, shifting your weight onto your front leg while keeping your back heel on the ground. You should feel a gentle stretch in your calf muscle.

5. **Hold the Stretch**: Hold the position for 15-30 seconds, maintaining a steady breath.

6. **Switch Legs**: Release the stretch and switch to the other leg, repeating the same steps.

7. **Repeat as Needed:** Perform the calf stretch 2-3 times on each leg to improve flexibility and reduce tightness in the calf muscles.

Safety Tips:
- **Avoid Bouncing:** Perform the stretch with slow, controlled movements. Bouncing can strain the muscles and increase the risk of injury.

- **Modify as Needed:** If you have difficulty maintaining balance, perform the stretch while seated on a chair with one leg extended at a time.

- **Consult a Professional:** If you have severe calf pain or a history of calf injuries, consult with a healthcare provider or physical therapist before performing calf stretches.

Incorporating the calf stretch into your regular routine can help maintain flexibility in your lower legs, improve circulation, and reduce discomfort associated with tight calf muscles.

Quadriceps Stretch

The quadriceps stretch is essential for improving flexibility in the front of the thigh and enhancing mobility. Follow these steps to perform the quadriceps stretch effectively:

1. **Stand Tall:** Stand upright with your feet hip-width apart and maintain good posture with your shoulders relaxed and spine straight.

2. **Hold onto Support**: Use a wall or sturdy chair for support if needed to maintain balance.

3. **Bend One Knee:** Bend your right knee and lift your right foot towards your buttocks, grasping your ankle or top of your foot with your right hand.

4. **Keep Knees Together:** Keep your knees close together. Avoid letting your knee move forward; instead, gently push your hip forward slightly to deepen the stretch.

5. **Feel the Stretch**: You should feel a gentle stretch along the front of your thigh and hip. Hold the position for 15-30 seconds.

6. **Maintain Breathing:** Breathe deeply and steadily throughout the stretch to help relax your muscles.

7. **Switch Legs:** Release the stretch and switch to the left leg, repeating the same steps.

8. **Repeat as Needed:** Perform the quadriceps stretch 2-3 times on each leg to improve flexibility and reduce tightness in the quadriceps muscles.

Safety Tips:
- **Avoid Overarching Your Back**: Keep your lower back in a neutral position and avoid arching it excessively during the stretch.

- **Use Support as Needed:** If balance is challenging, hold onto a chair or wall for support.

- **Modify as Needed:** If you have difficulty reaching your foot, use a strap or towel looped around your ankle to gently pull it towards your buttocks.

- **Consult a Professional:** If you have knee problems or hip issues, consult with a healthcare provider or physical therapist before performing quadriceps stretches.

Adding the quadriceps stretch into your routine can help maintain flexibility in your thighs, improve lower body mobility, and enhance overall comfort during daily activities.

Chapter 4: Full Body Stretches

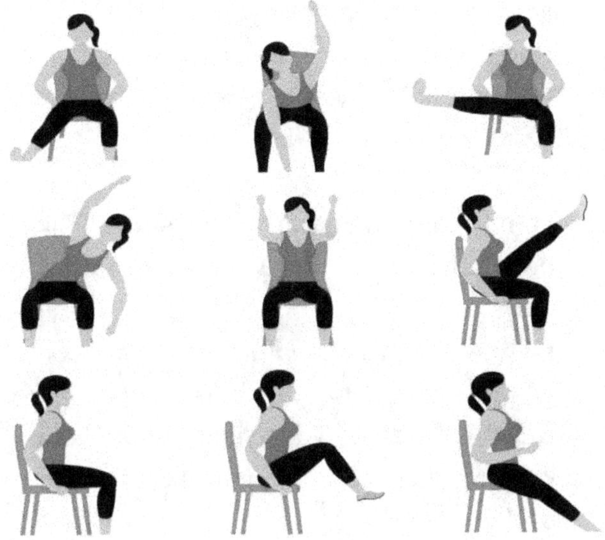

Seated Forward Bend

The seated forward bend is an effective stretch for improving flexibility in the hamstrings, lower back, and spine. It's especially suitable for seniors as it can be done comfortably while seated. Follow these steps to perform the seated forward bend safely and effectively:

1. **Sit Comfortably**: Sit on the edge of a sturdy chair with your feet flat on the floor, hip-width apart. Ensure your back is straight and shoulders are relaxed.

2. **Extend Your Legs**: If possible, extend your legs straight out in front of you with your heels on the floor and toes pointing upwards. If this is uncomfortable, you can keep your knees slightly bent.

3. **Inhale and Lengthen Your Spine**: Take a deep breath in and lengthen your spine, sitting up tall.

4. **Exhale and Lean Forward:** As you exhale, gently hinge at your hips and lean forward. Reach towards your feet with your hands, keeping your back straight. Avoid rounding your back.

5. **Go as Far as Comfortable:** Reach as far as comfortable without straining. You should feel a gentle stretch along your hamstrings and lower back. If you can't reach your feet, place your hands on your shins or knees.

6. **Hold the Stretch:** Hold the position for 15-30 seconds, breathing deeply and steadily.

7. **Return to Start:** Slowly rise back up to a seated position on an inhale, keeping your spine straight as you lift.

8. **Repeat as Needed**: Perform the seated forward bend 2-3 times to enhance flexibility and reduce tension in the back and legs.

Safety Tips:

- **Avoid Straining:** Only stretch to the point of mild tension or discomfort. Never push to the point of pain.

- **Maintain Proper Form:** Keep your back straight and hinge at the hips to avoid straining your lower back.

- **Modify as Needed:** If you have tight hamstrings or lower back issues, keep your knees slightly bent to reduce strain.

- **Use Props:** If reaching your feet is difficult, use a towel or yoga strap looped around your feet to assist with the stretch.

- **Consult a Professional:** If you have chronic back pain or any spinal issues, consult with a healthcare provider or physical therapist before performing forward bends.

Incorporating the seated forward bend into your regular routine can help improve flexibility in your hamstrings and lower back, enhance spinal mobility, and promote overall comfort and well-being.

Cat-Cow Stretch

The Cat-Cow stretch is an excellent exercise for seniors to improve flexibility and mobility in the spine, as well as to relieve tension in the back and neck. This gentle, flowing movement can be done on the floor or on a bed. Follow these steps for a safe and effective Cat-Cow stretch:

1. **Starting Position:** Begin on your hands and knees in a tabletop position. Ensure your wrists are directly under your shoulders and your knees are under your hips. Keep your back flat and your head in a neutral position, looking down at the floor.

2. **Cat Pose:**
   - **Exhale**: Slowly round your spine towards the ceiling, tucking your tailbone and chin towards your chest. Allow your head to drop, stretching the back of your neck.
   - **Hold for a moment**: Feel the stretch through your back.

3. **Cow Pose**:
   - **Inhale**: Arch your back, allowing your belly to sink towards the floor. Lift your head and tailbone towards the ceiling, looking slightly upward without straining your neck.
   - **Hold for a moment**: Feel the stretch through your abdomen and chest.

4. **Flow Between Poses**: Continue to flow between Cat and Cow poses, synchronizing your breath with your movements. Exhale as you move into Cat Pose and inhale as you move into Cow Pose.

5. **Repeat the Sequence**: Perform the Cat-Cow stretch for 1-2 minutes, moving smoothly and gently between each position.

Safety Tips:
- **Move Slowly:** Perform each movement slowly and with control to avoid straining your back or neck.

- **Breathe Deeply**: Synchronize your breath with your movements to maximize the benefits of the stretch.

- **Modify as Needed:** If you have wrist pain, try performing the stretch on your fists or forearms instead of your palms. Alternatively, you can do a seated version of Cat-Cow in a chair.

- **Listen to Your Body**: Only move within a range of motion that feels comfortable and pain-free. If you experience any discomfort, stop and consult with a healthcare professional.

Adding the Cat-Cow stretch to your routine can improve spinal flexibility, increase mobility, and reduce tension in your back and neck. This gentle exercise is particularly beneficial for seniors, promoting overall spinal health and well-being.

Chapter 5: Stretching Routines

Morning Routine

Starting your day with a morning stretching routine can set a positive tone for the rest of the day. For seniors a morning routine focused on gentle stretches can enhance flexibility, improve circulation, and reduce stiffness. Here's a suggested morning stretching routine to help you wake up your body and prepare for the day ahead:

1. **Neck Stretch:**
   - **Start Position:** Sit or stand tall, with your shoulders relaxed.
   - **Stretch:** Slowly tilt your head to one side, bringing your ear towards your shoulder. Hold for 15-30 seconds, then switch sides.
   - **Benefit**: Relieves tension in the neck and shoulders.

2. **Shoulder Stretch:**
   - **Start Position:** Stand or sit with your spine straight.

- Stretch: Reach one arm across your body and use your opposite hand to gently pull your arm towards your chest. Hold for 15-30 seconds, then switch sides.
  - **Benefit:** Improves flexibility and reduces stiffness in the shoulders.

3. **Chest Stretch:**
   - **Start Position:** Stand or sit upright with your hands clasped behind your back.
   - **Stretch**: Slowly lift your arms and gently squeeze your shoulder blades together, opening up your chest. Hold for 15-30 seconds.
   - **Benefit**: Enhances posture and relieves tension in the chest and shoulders.

4. **Seated Forward Bend**:
   - **Start Position**: Sit on the edge of a chair with your feet flat on the floor.
   - **Stretch**: Extend your legs straight out in front of you and hinge at your hips to lean forward, reaching towards your feet. Hold for 15-30 seconds.
   - **Benefit:** Stretches the hamstrings and lower back, improving flexibility.

5. **Cat-Cow Stretch:**
    - **Start Position:** Begin on your hands and knees in a tabletop position.
    - **Cat Pose:** Exhale and round your spine towards the ceiling, tucking your chin to your chest.
    - **Cow Pose**: Inhale and arch your back, lifting your head and tailbone towards the ceiling.
    - **Repeat**: Flow between Cat and Cow poses for 1-2 minutes.
    - **Benefit**: Increases spinal flexibility and relieves back tension.

6. **Quadriceps Stretch:**
    - **Start Position:** Stand tall, using a wall or chair for support.
    - **Stretch**: Bend one knee and bring your heel towards your buttocks, holding your ankle with your hand. Keep your knees close together. Hold for 15-30 seconds, **then switch sides.**
    - **Benefit**: Stretches the front of the thigh, improving lower body flexibility.

7. **Calf Stretch:**
    - **Start Position:** Stand facing a wall with your hands placed on the wall for support.

- **Stretch:** Step one foot back and press your heel into the ground while bending your front knee. Hold for 15-30 seconds, then switch sides.
  - **Benefit**: Improves flexibility in the calf muscles and enhances lower leg circulation.

8. **Hamstring Stretch:**
   - **Start Position**: Sit on the edge of a chair with one leg extended straight out.
   - **Stretch**: Lean forward from your hips, reaching towards your toes while keeping your back straight. Hold for 15-30 seconds, then switch sides.
   - **Benefit:** Enhances flexibility in the hamstrings and reduces lower back stiffness.

Safety Tips:

- **Move Gently**: Perform each stretch with slow, controlled movements to avoid injury.

- **Breathe Deeply:** Breathe deeply and steadily throughout each stretch to help relax your muscles.

- **Modify as Needed:** Adjust each stretch to your comfort level and use support if necessary.

- **Listen to Your Body**: Stop any stretch that causes pain and consult with a healthcare professional if needed.

Incorporating this morning routine into your daily schedule can help you start the day feeling more flexible, energized, and ready for the activities ahead.

Evening Routine

Ending your day with an evening stretching routine can help relax your muscles, reduce tension, and promote better sleep. For seniors, a gentle stretching routine in the evening can also improve overall flexibility and mobility. Here's a suggested evening stretching routine to help you unwind and prepare for a restful night:

1. **Neck Stretch:**
   - **Start Position:** Sit or stand tall, with your shoulders relaxed.
   - **Stretch**: Slowly tilt your head to one side, bringing your ear towards your shoulder. Hold for 15-30 seconds, then switch sides.

o   **Benefit**: Relieves tension in the neck and shoulders accumulated throughout the day.

2. **Shoulder Roll:**
    o   **Start Position:** Sit or stand with your spine straight.
    o   **Movement:** Roll your shoulders forward in a circular motion for 10-15 seconds, then roll them backward for another 10-15 seconds.
    o   **Benefit:** Loosens up tight shoulder muscles and improves circulation.

3. **Chest Stretch:**
    o   **Start Position**: Stand or sit upright with your hands clasped behind your back.
    o   **Stretch**: Slowly lift your arms and gently squeeze your shoulder blades together, opening up your chest. Hold for 15-30 seconds.
    o   **Benefit:** Opens up the chest and helps counteract poor posture.\

4. **Seated Forward Bend:**
    o   **Start Position:** Sit on the edge of a chair with your feet flat on the floor.

- o **Stretch**: Extend your legs straight out in front of you and hinge at your hips to lean forward, reaching towards your feet. Hold for 15-30 seconds.
- o **Benefit:** Stretches the hamstrings and lower back, easing tension.

5. **Cat-Cow Stretch:**
   - o **Start Position**: Begin on your hands and knees in a tabletop position.
   - o **Cat Pose**: Exhale and round your spine towards the ceiling, tucking your chin to your chest.
   - o **Cow Pose:** Inhale and arch your back, lifting your head and tailbone towards the ceiling.
   - o **Repeat:** Flow between Cat and Cow poses for 1-2 minutes.
   - o **Benefit:** Promotes spinal flexibility and relieves back tension.

6. **Hip Flexor Stretch:**
   - o **Start Position**: Stand or kneel on one knee, with the other foot in front, creating a 90-degree angle with both legs.
   - o **Stretch:** Push your hips gently forward while keeping your back straight. Hold for 15-30 seconds, then switch sides.

- o **Benefit**: Stretches the hip flexors and helps reduce lower back tension.

7. **Quadriceps Stretch:**
   - o **Start Position:** Stand tall, using a wall or chair for support.
   - o **Stretch:** Bend one knee and bring your heel towards your buttocks, holding your ankle with your hand. Keep your knees close together. Hold for 15-30 seconds, then switch sides.
   - o **Benefit**: Stretches the front of the thigh, promoting lower body relaxation.

8. **Calf Stretch:**
   - o **Start Position:** Stand facing a wall with your hands placed on the wall for support.
   - o **Stretch**: Step one foot back and press your heel into the ground while bending your front knee. Hold for 15-30 seconds, then switch sides.
   - o **Benefit:** Eases tension in the calf muscles and improves lower leg circulation.

9. **Hamstring Stretch:**
   - o **Start Position**: Sit on the edge of a chair with one leg extended straight out.

- o **Stretch:** Lean forward from your hips, reaching towards your toes while keeping your back straight. Hold for 15-30 seconds, then switch sides.
- o **Benefit:** Enhances flexibility in the hamstrings and reduces lower back stiffness.

10. Child's Pose:

- o **Start Position:** Kneel on the floor with your big toes touching and knees spread apart.
- o **Stretch:** Sit back on your heels and stretch your arms forward, lowering your chest towards the floor. Hold for 30 seconds to 1 minute.
- o **Benefit**: Relieves tension in the back, hips, and shoulders, promoting relaxation.

Safety Tips:
- **Move Gently:** Perform each stretch with slow, controlled movements to avoid injury.
- **Breathe Deeply:** Breathe deeply and steadily throughout each stretch to help relax your muscles.
- **Modify as Needed:** Adjust each stretch to your comfort level and use support if necessary.

- Listen to Your Body: Stop any stretch that causes pain and consult with a healthcare professional if needed.

Including this evening routine in your daily schedule can help you relax, reduce muscle tension, and prepare your body for a restful night's sleep.

Chair-based Routine

A chair-based stretching routine is perfect for seniors who may have mobility issues or prefer a seated exercise option. This routine focuses on improving flexibility, reducing stiffness, and enhancing overall mobility while using a sturdy chair for support.

1. **Neck Stretch:**
   - **Start Position:** Sit tall in a chair with your feet flat on the floor and your shoulders relaxed.
   - **Stretch**: Slowly tilt your head to one side, bringing your ear towards your shoulder. Hold for 15-30 seconds, then switch sides.
   - **Benefit**: Relieves tension in the neck and shoulders.

2. **Shoulder Stretch:**
   - **Start Position**: Sit with your spine straight and feet flat on the floor.
   - **Stretch:** Reach one arm across your body and use your opposite hand to gently pull your arm towards your chest. Hold for 15-30 seconds, then switch sides.
   - **Benefit:** Improves flexibility and reduces stiffness in the shoulders.

3. **Chest Stretch:**
   - **Start Position:** Sit upright with your hands clasped behind your back.
   - **Stretch**: Slowly lift your arms and gently squeeze your shoulder blades together, opening up your chest. Hold for 15-30 seconds.
   - **Benefit**: Enhances posture and relieves tension in the chest and shoulders.

4. **Seated Forward Bend:**
   - **Start Position:** Sit on the edge of the chair with your feet flat on the floor.
   - **Stretch:** Extend your legs straight out in front of you and hinge at your hips to lean forward, reaching towards your feet. Hold for 15-30 seconds.

- **Benefit:** Stretches the hamstrings and lower back, improving flexibility.

5. **Seated Cat-Cow Stretch:**
   - **Start Position:** Sit on the edge of the chair with your feet flat on the floor.
   - **Cat Pose:** Exhale and round your spine, tucking your chin to your chest.
   - **Cow Pose:** Inhale and arch your back, lifting your head and chest.
   - **Repeat:** Flow between Cat and Cow poses for 1-2 minutes.
   - **Benefit:** Promotes spinal flexibility and relieves back tension.

6. **Seated Hip Flexor Stretch:**
   - **Start Position:** Sit on the edge of the chair with your feet flat on the floor.
   - **Stretch:** Move one leg back, allowing the knee to bend and the foot to stay flat on the floor, while the other leg remains bent at a 90-degree angle. Hold for 15-30 seconds, then switch sides.
   - **Benefit:** Stretches the hip flexors and reduces lower back tension.

7. **Seated Quadriceps Stretch:**
   - **Start Position**: Sit sideways on the chair with one leg bent and the other leg extended back.
   - **Stretch**: Hold the back of the chair for support and gently pull your extended leg's ankle towards your buttocks. Hold for 15-30 seconds, then switch sides.
   - **Benefit:** Stretches the front of the thigh, promoting lower body relaxation.

8. **Seated Calf Stretch:**
   - **Start Position:** Sit on the edge of the chair with your feet flat on the floor.
   - **Stretch**: Extend one leg out and place the heel on the floor with toes pointing upwards. Lean forward slightly to deepen the stretch. Hold for 15-30 seconds, then switch sides.
   - **Benefit**: Eases tension in the calf muscles and improves lower leg circulation.

9. **Seated Hamstring Stretch:**
   - **Start Position**: Sit on the edge of the chair with one leg extended straight out.
   - **Stretch:** Lean forward from your hips, reaching towards your toes while keeping

your back straight. Hold for 15-30 seconds, then switch sides.

- **Benefit:** Enhances flexibility in the hamstrings and reduces lower back stiffness.

10. Seated Side Stretch:

- **Start Position:** Sit upright with your feet flat on the floor.
- **Stretch:** Extend one arm overhead and gently lean to the opposite side, feeling the stretch along your side. Hold for 15-30 seconds, then switch sides.
- **Benefit**: Stretches the sides of your torso, enhancing flexibility and relieving tension.

Safety Tips:

- **Move Gently**: Perform each stretch with slow, controlled movements to avoid injury.
- **Breathe Deeply:** Breathe deeply and steadily throughout each stretch to help relax your muscles.
- **Modify as Needed**: Adjust each stretch to your comfort level and use support if necessary.
- Listen to Your Body: Stop any stretch that causes pain and consult with a healthcare professional if needed.

Incorporating this chair-based routine into your daily schedule can help you improve flexibility, reduce muscle stiffness, and enhance overall comfort and well-being.

Chapter 6: Additional Tips

Incorporating Stretching into Daily Life

Incorporating stretching into your daily life is essential for maintaining flexibility, reducing stiffness, and promoting overall well-being, especially for seniors. By making stretching a regular part of your routine, you can enhance your mobility, improve your posture, and reduce the risk of injuries. Here are some practical ways to integrate stretching into your everyday activities:

1. **Morning Routine:**
   - **Start Your Day Right:** Begin each day with a gentle morning stretch routine to wake up your muscles and joints. Simple stretches such as neck stretches, shoulder rolls, and seated forward bends can help you feel more flexible and energized.
   - **Consistency is Key:** Make it a habit to spend 5-10 minutes stretching every morning. This sets a positive tone for the rest of your day.

2. **Work Breaks:**
   - o **Micro-breaks:** Take short breaks during your work or daily activities to stand up and stretch. This is particularly important if you spend long periods sitting.
   - o **Stretch at Your Desk:** Incorporate seated stretches such as seated cat-cow stretches, seated side stretches, and ankle rolls while working at your desk.

3. **Television Time:**
   - o **Stretch While Watching TV:** Use commercial breaks or downtime while watching TV to perform a few stretches. This can include seated hamstring stretches, seated calf stretches, or gentle spinal twists.
   - o **Multitask:** Keep a yoga mat or a comfortable chair nearby to stretch while enjoying your favorite shows.

4. **Evening Routine:**
   - o **Wind Down:** End your day with a relaxing evening stretch routine. Incorporate stretches such as the seated forward bend, cat-cow stretch, and child's pose to help your body relax and prepare for sleep.

- Promote Relaxation: Gentle stretches in the evening can also help reduce tension and promote a more restful night's sleep.

5. **Incorporate into Daily Tasks:**
   - **Stretch While Cooking**: Use time spent waiting for water to boil or food to cook as an opportunity to do a few stretches. For example, perform calf stretches or hip flexor stretches.
   - **Household Chores:** Integrate stretches into household chores. For instance, after vacuuming or sweeping, do a standing quadriceps stretch or a chest stretch.

6. **Use Technology:**
   - **Reminders:** Set reminders on your phone or use a stretching app to prompt you to stretch throughout the day.
   - **Follow Online Guides:** Utilize online videos or guides that offer stretching routines tailored for seniors to keep your routine varied and engaging.

7. **Social Stretching:**
   - **Group Activities**: Join a stretching class or a yoga group for seniors. The social

aspect can make stretching more enjoyable and keep you motivated.

- o Stretch with a Friend: Invite a friend or family member to stretch with you. This can be a fun way to stay committed to your stretching routine.

8. Adapt Stretches to Your Needs:

- o **Customize**: Tailor your stretching routine to suit your individual needs and limitations. Focus on areas where you feel the most tension or stiffness.
- o **Listen to Your Body:** Pay attention to your body's signals and adjust your stretches accordingly. Never push yourself to the point of pain.

Safety Tips:

- **Move Gently:** Perform each stretch with slow, controlled movements to avoid injury.
- **Breathe Deeply**: Breathe deeply and steadily throughout each stretch to help relax your muscles.
- **Modify as Needed:** Adjust each stretch to your comfort level and use support if necessary.
- **Consult a Professional:** If you have any health concerns or chronic conditions, consult with a

healthcare provider or physical therapist before starting a new stretching routine.

Integrating stretching into your daily life can significantly improve your flexibility, mobility, and overall quality of life. With these practical tips, you can easily make stretching a regular and enjoyable part of your daily routine.

Staying Consistent

Maintaining consistency in your stretching routine is crucial for reaping the long-term benefits of improved flexibility, reduced stiffness, and overall well-being. For seniors, developing and sticking to a regular stretching regimen can enhance your quality of life and help you stay active and independent. Here are some strategies to help you stay consistent with your stretching exercises:

1. **Set Realistic Goals:**
   - **Start Small**: Begin with short, manageable sessions of 5-10 minutes each day and gradually increase the duration as you become more comfortable.
   - **Be Specific**: Set clear, achievable goals such as stretching for 10 minutes every

morning or incorporating three stretching breaks into your day.

2. **Create a Routine:**
    - **Same Time, Same Place:** Designate specific times of the day for stretching, such as first thing in the morning and before bed. Having a consistent schedule helps establish a habit.
    - **Use Cues:** Associate stretching with daily activities, like stretching after brushing your teeth or during TV commercials, to create a natural reminder

3. **Track Your Progress:**
    - **Keep a Journal:** Record your stretching activities in a journal to monitor your progress and stay motivated.
    - **Celebrate Milestones**: Acknowledge and celebrate small achievements, such as increased flexibility or completing a full week of stretching.

4. **Stay Motivated:**
    - **Enjoyable Routine:** Choose stretches that you enjoy and that make you feel good. This will make you more likely to stick with your routine.

- Involve Others: Stretch with a friend, family member, or join a class. Social interaction can make the activity more enjoyable and keep you accountable.

5. **Use Technology:**
   - **Set Reminders:** Use your phone or a stretching app to set reminders and alerts to prompt you to stretch.
   - **Follow Online Programs**: Engage with online stretching programs or videos designed for seniors to keep your routine varied and interesting.

6. **Adapt to Your Lifestyle:**
   - **Be Flexible:** If you miss a session, don't get discouraged. Simply resume your routine as soon as possible.
   - **Integrate Into Daily Life**: Incorporate stretching into everyday activities, such as while waiting for the kettle to boil or after gardening.

7. **Mind Your Body:**
   - **Listen to Your Body**: Pay attention to how your body feels during and after stretching. Adjust the intensity and duration based on your comfort level.

o   Rest When Needed: If you feel pain or excessive discomfort, take a break and allow your body to rest.

8. **Seek Professional Guidance:**
    o   **Consult Experts:** If you're unsure about your stretching technique or routine, seek advice from a physical therapist or fitness professional.
    o   **Regular Check-Ins:** Periodically review your progress and routine with a professional to ensure you're on the right track.

Practical Tips for Consistency:
- **Visual Reminders**: Place notes or visual cues around your home to remind you to stretch.
- **Comfortable Environment**: Create a dedicated, comfortable space for stretching with a mat and any necessary props.
- **Positive Reinforcement**: Reward yourself for staying consistent, whether it's a small treat or a relaxing activity you enjoy.

By incorporating these strategies, you can develop a consistent and effective stretching routine that fits seamlessly into your daily life. Regular stretching will help you maintain flexibility, reduce stiffness, and enhance your overall health and well-being, allowing you to stay active and independent for years to come.

Combining Stretching with Other Exercises

Integrating stretching with other forms of exercise can create a well-rounded fitness routine that enhances overall health, flexibility, and strength. For seniors, combining stretching with aerobic, strength, and balance exercises can optimize physical fitness and improve daily functioning. Here's how to effectively incorporate stretching into a comprehensive exercise regimen:

1. **Before Exercise: Dynamic Stretching**

   - **Warm-Up Routine:** Begin with dynamic stretches that gently prepare your muscles for more intense activity. Dynamic stretching involves controlled movements that gradually increase your range of motion.
   - **Examples:** Arm circles, leg swings, and walking lunges can help increase blood flow and improve flexibility.

2. **During Exercise: Active Stretching**
   - o **Incorporate Stretching:** Include active stretching within your workout. For example, after a set of strength exercises, perform a related stretch to keep muscles flexible and reduce stiffness.
   - o **Examples:** After a set of squats, perform a quadriceps stretch; after upper body exercises, stretch the chest and shoulders.

3. **After Exercise: Static Stretching**
   - o **Cool-Down Routine:** Conclude your workout with static stretching to help relax muscles and improve flexibility. Static stretching involves holding a stretch for 15-30 seconds without movement.
   - o **Examples:** Hamstring stretches, calf stretches, and seated forward bends can help reduce muscle tension and aid recovery.

4. **Combining with Aerobic Exercise**
   - o **Walking or Jogging:** Begin with a warm-up that includes dynamic stretching. After your aerobic session, perform static stretches to help relax muscles and prevent stiffness.

- **Example Routine**: Start with leg swings and arm circles before walking. After your walk, perform calf stretches, hamstring stretches, and a seated forward bend.

5. **Combining with Strength Training**
    - **Pre-Workout:** Warm up with dynamic stretches targeting the muscle groups you will work on.
    - **Intra-Workout:** Perform active stretches between sets to maintain flexibility.
    - **Post-Workout:** Finish with static stretches to enhance muscle recovery and flexibility.
    - **Example Routine**: Warm up with walking lunges and arm swings. Between sets of weightlifting, do shoulder stretches. After the session, stretch your chest, quads, and hamstrings.

6. **Combining with Balance Exercises**
    - **Yoga and Tai Chi:** Both yoga and Tai Chi integrate stretching with balance and strength exercises, promoting flexibility, stability, and relaxation.

- **Daily Practice:** Incorporate yoga or Tai Chi sessions into your weekly routine for a holistic approach to fitness.
- **Example Routine:** Include yoga poses like downward dog, warrior pose, and cat-cow stretches to enhance flexibility and balance.

Practical Tips for Integration:

- **Plan Your Routine:** Schedule specific times for stretching within your workout plan. This helps ensure that you consistently include stretching in your fitness regimen.

- **Balanced Approach**: Aim for a balanced routine that includes a mix of stretching, aerobic, strength, and balance exercises to cover all aspects of physical fitness.

- **Adjust Intensity:** Modify the intensity and duration of stretching based on the type and intensity of the other exercises you are performing.

- **Stay Hydrated:** Drink plenty of water before, during, and after exercising to keep your muscles hydrated and reduce the risk of cramps.

- **Listen to Your Body**: Pay attention to how your body responds to the combined exercises. Adjust your routine as needed to avoid overexertion and injury.

Safety Tips:
- **Warm Up Properly**: Always start with a warm-up to prepare your muscles for more intense activity and reduce the risk of injury.
- **Focus on Form**: Use proper form for all stretches and exercises to maximize benefits and minimize the risk of injury.
- **Avoid Overstretching:** Stretch to the point of mild tension, not pain. Overstretching can lead to muscle strain or injury.
- **Consult a Professional:** If you're unsure about combining stretching with other exercises, seek guidance from a fitness professional or physical therapist.

By combining stretching with other types of exercises, you can create a comprehensive fitness routine that enhances flexibility, strength, balance, and overall health. This integrated approach helps ensure that you stay active, mobile, and independent, supporting a higher quality of life.

Conclusion

Incorporating regular stretching into your daily routine offers a wealth of advantages. Stretching enhances flexibility, allowing for greater ease of movement in everyday activities. It alleviates muscle tension and stiffness, promoting a sense of relaxation and well-being.

By improving circulation, stretching supports overall cardiovascular health and aids in the recovery process after physical activity. Additionally, consistent stretching helps maintain proper posture, reduces the risk of injuries, and can even alleviate chronic pain in areas such as the back, neck, and shoulders.

Your commitment to a regular stretching routine is a powerful step toward maintaining and enhancing your physical health. It's never too late to start, and every little bit counts. By staying active and integrating stretching into your daily life, you're investing in your future mobility and independence. Remember, the key is consistency. Make stretching a natural part of your morning and evening routines, incorporate it into your daily activities, and combine it with other forms of exercise for a well-rounded fitness regimen.

Your body will thank you for the care and attention you provide through these gentle movements. So, keep moving, stay flexible, and continue to enjoy the many benefits that come with a dedicated stretching practice. Here's to a healthier, more active you in your golden years.

Appendix

Glossary of Terms

To aid in your understanding of stretching exercises and fitness terminology, here are some key terms frequently used throughout this guide:

1. **Dynamic Stretching**: Stretching exercises that involve continuous movement and are typically performed as part of a warm-up routine to prepare the muscles for physical activity.

2. **Static Stretching:** Stretching exercises that involve holding a stretch position for a period of time (usually 15-30 seconds) without movement, aimed at improving flexibility and reducing muscle tension.

3. **Flexibility**: The ability of muscles and joints to move through their full range of motion without discomfort or restriction.

4. **Range of Motion (ROM):** The extent to which a joint can move in various directions, including flexion, extension, abduction, and adduction.

5. **Mobility**: The ability to move freely and easily, encompassing both flexibility and joint function.

6. **Muscle Stiffness:** A sensation of resistance or tightness in muscles, often due to prolonged immobility or physical exertion.

7. **Posture:** The alignment of the body parts in relation to one another while standing, sitting, or lying down. Good posture helps prevent strain on muscles and joints.

8. **Warm-Up:** Gentle exercises performed before a workout or physical activity to prepare the body by increasing heart rate, circulation, and flexibility.

9. **Cool-Down:** Gentle exercises or stretching performed after a workout or physical activity to gradually decrease heart rate, prevent muscle soreness, and promote relaxation.

10. **Balance Exercises:** Activities designed to improve stability and prevent falls by enhancing proprioception (awareness of body position) and strengthening muscles involved in maintaining balance.

11. **Aerobic Exercise:** Physical activity that increases heart rate and oxygen consumption over an extended period, such as walking, swimming, or cycling, to improve cardiovascular health.

12. **Strength Training:** Exercises using resistance (e.g., weights, resistance bands) to strengthen muscles, improve muscle tone, and enhance overall physical strength.

13. **Proprioception:** The body's ability to sense its position and movement in space, crucial for balance, coordination, and efficient movement.

14. **Physical Fitness**: Overall health and well-being achieved through regular physical activity, including cardiovascular endurance, muscular strength, flexibility, and balance.

15. **Chronic Pain:** Persistent pain lasting for weeks, months, or years, often associated with conditions like arthritis or back pain.

9 7 9 8 3 0 2 2 1 6 5 9 5